Nephrology Formulas

The Nephrology formula is designed to provide a tutored approach for Medical students, Residents, Attending physicians and other health care workers, to identify the various presentations of acid base disorders and other renal related calculations
A step by step integrated approach to acid base disorders provide a fast, simple and effective way to analysis of patient laboratory values
The formulas have been highlighted and presented in an easy to understand pattern. Complex formulas has been relevant to routine clinical care has been analyzed and constructed into easy to understand illustrations

The nephrology formula completed with examples is perfect for any health care practitioner involved in daily calculations of many of the regular nephrology related cases.

The pocket-fit size provide an appraised method of information easily available during rounds

The bases for identifying commonly questions asked in examinations has been revised and discussed here. Sample examples are presented in a simplified format.

Formulas in dialysis have been included for medical practitioners involved in calculations of dialysis related problems.

Compiled and Authored by

**Ebima Clifford Okundaye MD, FACP**

Consultant Nephrologist
Altru Health System,
Grand Forks, ND
Clinical Assistant Professor of Medicine
University of North Dakota Medical School
Grand Forks, ND

## TABLE OF CONTENTS            PAGES

**Acid – Base balance disorders**      **5**
- *Steps in acid base disorders (6-37)*
- *Anion gap calculation (21)*
- *Calculation of bicarbonate deficit (26)*
- *Urine anion gap (28)*
- *Metabolic Alkalosis (31)*
- *Respiratory acidosis and alkalosis (31)*
- *Metabolic acidosis in chronic kidney disease (37)*

**Body compartments volume calculations**      **38**
- Extracellular and intracellular volumes (39)
- Plasma water and blood volume (39-41)

**Electrolytes and water balance calculation**      **42**
- Correction of hyponatremia (47)
- Free water clearance calculation (49)
- Correction of hypernatremia (56)
- Fractional excretion of electrolytes (60)

**Acute renal failure, Chronic kidney disease And Nutrition in renal failure**      **67**
- Calculation of Estimated glomerular rates (71)
- Calorie and protein prescription in renal failure (74)

**Dialysis related formulas**      **77**
*Dialysis adequacy - Peritoneal dialysis clearance (78)*
*Residual renal function (79)*
*Hemodialysis ( 80 )and CRRT clearance (82-83)*
*Plasma exchange volumes (86)*

**Case practice questions and answers**      **88**

# Chapter 1

## ACID BASE BALANCE DISORDERS

**Normal ranges of values**

| | | **Units** |
|---|---|---|
| Sodium | 136 - 145 | mmol/L |
| Potassium | 3.5 - 5.1 | mmol/L |
| Chloride | 98 - 107 | mmol/L |
| BUN, Bld | 7 - 22 | mg/dL |
| Creatinine | 0.6 - 1.3 | mg/dl |
| Glucose | 70 - 99 | mg/dL |
| Calcium | 8.5 - 10.1 | mg/dL |
| Phosphorus | 2.5 - 4.9 | mg/dL |
| Albumin | 3.4 - 5.0 | g/dL |
| CO2 or HCO3 | 21.0 - 32.0 | mmol/L |

*All values for electrolytes given in this book are assumed measured in the standard units given above*

1  Henderson-Hasselbalch equation:

$$pH = 6.10 + \log([HCO_3^-] \div [0.03 \times PCO_2])$$

Where pH – arterial pH or venous pH + 0.03

HC03- serum bicarbonate value

PCO2- partial pressure of carbon dioxide

## Using this equation

To obtain Normal serum pH

Given normal PCO2 range 40-44 and serum HC03 range 24-26

$$PH = 6.1 + \log\left\{\frac{[24]}{(0.03 \times 40)}\right\}$$

$$= 6.1 + \log 24/1.2$$
$$= 6.1 + \log 20$$
$$= 6.1 + 1.3$$
$$= 7.40$$

Usually normal range though varies from 7.37 - 7.40

II

## STEPS TO IDENTYFING ALL ACID- BASE DISORDERS

# STEP 1

Identify the major acid base disorder

Acidosis = Any PH < 7.37 regardless of serum HCO3

Alkalosis – Any PH  > 7.40 regardless of serum HCO3

### Metabolic acidosis

pH < 7.40 AND  serum HC03 < 24

Divided into 2 types

- Anion gap metabolic acidosis (addition of acid as H+)

-Non anion gap metabolic acidosis   (primary loss of Bicarbonate without in generation of H+, thereby occurs only in renal loss as RTA or GI colon loss as diarrhea

### Metabolic alkalosis

pH >7.40 AND serum HC03>24

### Respiratory acidosis

pH <7.4 AND serum Hc03 > 24    with PCO2 > 45mmhg

### Respiratory alkalosis

PH>7.4 AND serum HC03 <24   with PC02 <45mmhg

*Note a low serum HC03 alone does not necessarily mean metabolic acidosis. It can also be an alkalosis. So you need the pH always.*

## III

## Analyzing arterial blood gas (ABG) report

| | |
|---|---|
| **pH** | **7.37** |
| **PCO2** | **45** |
| **PO2** | **90** |
| **HCO3** | **23** |

Any pH <7.37 is suggestive of acidosis while a pH >7.40 is suggestive of alkalosis. Any value within 7.37-7.40 can be normal or alkalosis

The arterial pH is the standard, but in the absence of an arterial blood gas, the arterial pH can be calculated from a venous blood gas sample by

## Arterial pH = Venous pH + 0.03

*The arterial sample HC03 level is calculated from the arterial pC02 and p02 levels and not actually measured like the serum HC03 in the Basic metabolic panel (BMP).. Thus the ABG HC03 level is not real and should not be use in any calculation. Always use the BMP HC03 level.*

## IV

## Common causes of Acidosis

### *Non-Anion Gap*

Diarrhea
Renal Tubular acidosis
Renal failure

### *Anion Gap Metabolic acidosis*

Lactic acidosis
Ketoacidosis- Diabetic
       - Alcohol
       - Fasting
Ingestion – methanol, ethylene glycol, ethanol, Salicylate poisoning
Renal failure- mostly chronic
Pyroglutamic acidosis

## Case Practice

### A-1

77 yr old male with hypertension, remote history of tobacco use admitted now for abdominal pain, patient clinically appears septic with hypotension, lab studies shows

| | |
|---|---|
| Sodium | 144 |
| Chloride | 89 |
| Bicarbonate | 33 |
| Albumin | 3.8 |
| **Potassium** | **3.5** |
| **Calcium** | **9.0** |
| **Creatinine** | **1.3** |
| **Blood urea** | **30** |

### What is the acid base disorder?

1. There is a high bicarbonate( $HCO_3$) level – suggesting a possible metabolic alkalosis, But since high bicarbonate level can also be found in respiratory acidosis, the arterial PH is needed to identify the primary disorder

Further laboratory test with arterial blood gas shows

| | |
|---|---|
| pH | 7.45 |
| $PCO_2$ | 49 |
| $PO_2$ | 92 |
| $HCO_3$ | 25 |

In this ABG result the primary disorder is Alkalosis
And since there is elevated serum bicarbonate level, then the disorder is *Primary Metabolic alkalosis*

### A-2

45 year old Caucasian female with history of diabetes mellitus, history of peripheral vascular disease and hypertension. She was seen for chronic diarrhea. Her laboratory tests shows

Sodium 138
Chloride 98
Bicarbonate 29
Albumin 3.8
**Potassium 3.4**
**Calcium 9.0**

*Arterial blood gas analysis shows*
pH 7.41
PCO2 49
PO2 95
HCO3 25

### What is the primary acid base disorder?

1 Since high serum bicarbonate level – suggest either a primary metabolic alkalosis or a respiratory acidosis

2 However the high arterial PH of 7.40 is consistent with an alkalotic state.

Thus the patient has **a primary metabolic alkalosis**

### A-3

**A** 23 yr old female with depression have the following labs

Sodium 136
Chloride 98
Bicarbonate 20
Albumin 3.8
Potassium 3.5
Calcium 9.0
Creatinine 1.3
Blood urea 30

Arterial blood gas
pH        7.40
HCO3      19
PCO2      32

What is the primary acid base disorder?

1 Since low serum bicarbonate level – suggestive either a primary metabolic acidosis or a respiratory alkalosis

2 However the high arterial PH of 7.40 is consistent with an alkalotic state.

Thus the patient has **a primary respiratory alkalosis**

### A- 4

45 year old Caucasian female with Crohn's disease admitted for weakness, recent onset of diarrhea. Her laboratory tests shows

| | |
|---|---|
| Sodium | 129 |
| Chloride | 102 |
| Bicarbonate | 17 |
| Albumin | 3.8 |
| **Potassium** | **3.1** |
| **Calcium** | **9.0** |

*Arterial blood gas analysis shows*

| | |
|---|---|
| pH | 7.23 |
| PC02 | 44 |
| P02 | 90 |
| HC03 | 25 |

1 Since low serum bicarbonate level – suggesting either a primary metabolic acidosis or a respiratory alkalosis
2 However the low arterial PH of 7.23 is consistent with an acidosis state.

Thus the patient has **a primary metabolic acidosis (hyperchloremic non anion gap acidosis)**

## A- 5

58 year old female with history of seizure disorder on acetazolamide, seen in the hospital post fall at home. Her laboratory tests shows

| | |
|---|---|
| Sodium | 134 |
| Chloride | 102 |
| Bicarbonate | 17 |
| Albumin | 3.8 |
| **Potassium** | **3.6** |
| **Calcium** | **8.5** |

*Arterial blood gas analysis shows*
| | |
|---|---|
| pH | 7.31 |
| $PCO_2$ | 35 |
| $PO_2$ | 90 |
| $HCO_3$ | 18 |

= Primary metabolic acidosis

## A-6

A 65 year old male with history of mental retardation, schizophrenia prior lithium use admitted for weakness. His laboratory tests shows

| | |
|---|---|
| Sodium | 137 |
| Chloride | 112 |
| Bicarbonate | 20.4 |
| Albumin | 3.8 |
| Potassium | 3.7 |
| Calcium | 8.9 |
| BUN | 56 |
| Creatinine | 2.9 |

*Arterial blood gas analysis shows*
| | |
|---|---|
| pH | 7.27 |
| $PCO_2$ | 56 |
| $PO_2$ | 90 |
| $HCO_3$ | 56 |

1 Since low serum bicarbonate level – suggestive of either a primary metabolic acidosis or a respiratory alkalosis

2 However the low arterial PH of 7.27 is consistent with an acidosis state.

Thus the patient has **a primary metabolic acidosis (Actually a combined metabolic and respiratory acidosis)**

### A-7

**24 yr old female admitted for suicide attempt with aspirin overdose. Her** laboratory tests shows

| | |
|---|---|
| Sodium | 136 |
| Chloride | 92 |
| Bicarbonate | 20 |
| Albumin | 3.8 |
| Potassium | 3.5 |
| Calcium | 8.9 |

*Arterial blood gas analysis shows*
| | |
|---|---|
| pH | 7.42 |
| PCO2 | 23 |
| PO2 | 90 |
| HCO3 | 23 |

1 Since low serum bicarbonate level – suggestive of either a primary metabolic acidosis or a respiratory alkalosis

2 However the high arterial PH of 7.42 is consistent with an alkalosis state.

Thus the patient has **a primary respiratory alkalosis**

## A-8

44 yr old female with schizophrenia and history of seizure disorder. Her laboratory tests shows

| | |
|---|---|
| Sodium | 140 |
| Chloride | 99 |
| Bicarbonate | 18 |
| Albumin | 3.8 |
| Potassium | 3.7 |
| Calcium | 8.9 |

*Arterial blood gas analysis shows*

| | |
|---|---|
| pH | 7.35 |
| PCO2 | 40 |
| PO2 | 80 |
| HCO3 | 40 |

1 Since low serum bicarbonate level indicates either a primary metabolic acidosis or a respiratory alkalosis

2 However the low arterial PH of 7.18 is consistent with an acidosis state.

Thus the patient has **a primary metabolic acidosis**

## A-9

A 67 yr old male with COPD, on home oxygen, admitted for shortness of breath. She was noted with respiratory wheeze. Her laboratory tests shows

| | |
|---|---|
| Sodium | 138 |
| Chloride | 100 |
| Bicarbonate | 34 |
| Albumin | 3.8 |
| Potassium | 4.5 |
| Calcium | 8.9 |

*Arterial blood gas analysis shows*
pH        7.34
PCO2      68
PO2       62
HCO3      56


1 Since high serum bicarbonate level –either a primary metabolic alkalosis or a respiratory acidosis

2 However the low arterial PH of 7.34 is borderline for an acidotic state.

Thus the patient has **a primary respiratory acidosis**


### A-10

35 yr old male with acute onset diarrhea. A diagnosis of presumed gastroenteritis is made. His laboratory tests shows

Sodium       141
Chloride     109
Bicarbonate  19
Albumin      3.8
Potassium    3.4
Calcium      8.9
BUN          56
Creatinine   2.0

*Arterial blood gas analysis shows*
pH        7.36
PCO2      32
PO2       90
HCO3      33


1 Since low serum bicarbonate level – suggest either a primary metabolic acidosis or a respiratory alkalosis

2 However the low arterial PH of 7.36 is consistent with an acidosis state.

Thus the patient has **a primary metabolic acidosis**

### A-11

59 yr old male, with recent significant ibuprofen use for arthritis, is admitted for heartburn, nausea, or vomiting. His laboratory tests shows

| | |
|---|---|
| Sodium | 140 |
| Chloride | 112 |
| Bicarbonate | 29 |
| Albumin | 3.8 |
| Potassium | 3.0 |
| Calcium | 8.9 |

*Arterial blood gas analysis shows*

| | |
|---|---|
| pH | 7.42 |
| PCO2 | 33 |
| PO2 | 76 |

Since high serum bicarbonate level and high PH

Thus the patient has **a primary metabolic alkalosis**

### A-12

54 yr old male with multiple myeloma on chemotherapy seen in routine office visit. His laboratory tests shows

| | |
|---|---|
| Sodium | 140 |
| Chloride | 112 |
| Bicarbonate | 20 |
| Albumin | 3.8 |
| Potassium | 3.9 |
| Calcium | 8.9 |

*Arterial blood gas analysis shows*

pH 7.35
PCO2 41
PO2 76

A low serum bicarbonate level and low arterial PH of 7.27 is consistent with an acidotic state from a metabolic disorder

Thus the patient has **a primary metabolic acidosis**

# STEP 2

In metabolic Acidosis

## Evaluate for appropriate compensation

Calculating for respiratory compensation in metabolic acidosis

### 3 methods

A  Winters formula

  $PCO_2 = 1.5 (HCO_3) + 8 \pm 2$

B  $\Delta PCO_2 = 1.3 \times \Delta HCO_3$

C  $PCO_2$ = last 2 digits of pH

The Winters formula **is the most important and only one you need to know**

The third formula can be use as a quick glance for screening. But it does not give more information after that.

Interpretation of the Winters formula - if the calculated $PCO_2$ is within $\pm 2$ of the actual $PCO_2$ then there is a well respiratory compensated metabolic acidosis.

When the calculated $PCO_2$ is more than 2 above the provided $PCO_2$ then there is a secondary respiratory acidosis

if the $PCO_2$ is more than 2 below the provided $PCO_2$ then there is a secondary respiratory alkalosis

*Remember:*
*1. Winters formula is only use in metabolic acidosis*
*2. When applying the formula, there is no $\Delta$ calculation, you don't need to subtract the $PCO_2$ or $HCO_3$ from the normal value. Just simply use the numbers provided*

**Case Practice**

B-1

77 yr old male with hypertension and a remote history of tobacco use , is admitted now for pneumonia. He clinically appears septic with hypotension. His lab studies shows

| | |
|---|---|
| Sodium | 136 |
| Chloride | 97 |
| Bicarbonate | 18 |
| Albumin | 3.7 |
| **Potassium** | **4.1** |
| **Calcium** | **9.0** |

Arterial Blood gas shows

| | |
|---|---|
| pH | 7.34 |
| PCO2 | 40 |
| PO2 | 92 |
| HCO3 | 22 |

**Is the respiratory compensation adequate?**

1 There is a low bicarbonate (HCO3) level and a low arterial pH – suggesting a primary metabolic acidosis

Applying Winters formula

$PCO2 = 1.5 (HCO3) + 8 \pm 2$

$= 1.5 \times 18 + 8$

$= 27 + 8$

$= 35 \pm 2$

Therefore expected PCO2 is between 33 to 35

Since patient PCO2 is greater than expected of 35 then there is associated respiratory acidosis

B-2

77 yr old male with hypertension, remote history of Tobacco use admitted now for pneumonia, patient clinically appears dehydrated, lab studies shows

| | |
|---|---|
| Sodium | 136 |
| Chloride | 97 |
| Bicarbonate | 34 |
| Albumin | 3.7 |
| **Potassium** | **4.1** |
| **Calcium** | **9.0** |

Further laboratory test with arterial blood gas shows

| | |
|---|---|
| pH | 7.39 |
| $PCO_2$ | 60 |
| $PO_2$ | 92 |
| $HCO_3$ | 22 |

In this case the primary disorder is Alkalosis

And since there is also an elevated serum bicarbonate level, then the disorder is *Primary Metabolic alkalosis*

*To assess for respiratory compensation, we need to utilize respiratory changes for metabolic alkalosis as explained later.*
*Winters formula cannot be used here since it is metabolic alkalosis and not metabolic acidosis*


B-3

45 year old Caucasian female with history of Diabetes mellitus, Peripheral vascular disease and Hypertension. She was seen for chronic diarrhea. Her laboratory tests shows

| | |
|---|---|
| Sodium | 138 |
| Chloride | 98 |
| Bicarbonate | 21 |
| Albumin | 3.8 |
| **Potassium** | **3.4** |
| **Calcium** | **9.0** |

*Arterial blood gas analysis shows*
```
pH          7.32
PCO2        49
PO2         92
HCO3        25
```

## What is the primary acid base disorder?

1. Since low serum bicarbonate level – suggestive of either a primary metabolic acidosis or a respiratory alkalosis

2. The arterial PH of 7.34 is consistent with an acidotic state.

Thus the patient has **a primary metabolic acidosis**


To calculate for adequacy of compensation, we can apply the **Winters formula** here

PCO2 = 1.5 (HCO3) + 8 ± 2

Expected PCO2 =  1.5 × 21  + 8

$\quad\quad\quad\quad\quad\quad$ =   31 + 8

$\quad\quad\quad\quad\quad\quad$ = 39

Expected PCO2 = 39 ± 2

Since Actual PCO2 ( 49 ) is higher than Expected PCO2( 37-41), there is associated respiratory acidosis

## Thus the patient has both a metabolic acidosis and a respiratory acidosis

*So the winter formula can only identify 2 acid base disorders. That is a primary metabolic acidosis and presence of either a superimposed respiratory acidosis or alkalosis. It cannot tell if there is a third acid base disorder. Which at this time can either be a superimposed metabolic alkalosis or an additional type of metabolic acidosis to the primary one?*

To calculate for a third base disorder, we need anion gap calculation

**STEP 3**

**Identify presence of an increase in the Anion gap**

Calculate serum anion gap

### *SERUM ANION GAP (AG)*

Serum AG = Measured cations - measured anions

Since sodium (Na) is the primary measured cation and chloride (Cl) and bicarbonate (HCO3) are the primary measured anions.

Serum AG = Na - (Cl + HCO3)

Normal anion gap is 10-12

**STEP 4**

**Adjust the anion gap for serum albumin**

Serum albumin contributes to the Anion gap. Anion gap increase by 3.5 for every decrease in serum albumin below 4

**Actual anion GAP = Δ albumin x calculated anion gap**

Anion gap > 12 suggest an anion gap metabolic acidosis, if < 12 then it is normal anion gap metabolic acidosis

*Remember- 1. Anion gap calculation is only important in metabolic acidosis.*
*2. Lactate contribute 1:1 to increase in anion gap*

## STEP 5

Identify Anion gap relationship to serum HC03

The difference from the actual anion gap calculated (after correction for albumin) and the normal anion gap of 12 is called the change in anion gap (Δ Anion gap)

**Δ Anion gap = Calculated Anion gap - 12**

In Anion gap metabolic acidosis, due to the addition of H+, the level of decrease in serum HC03 correspond to the level of increase in anion gap.

So the change in Anion gap (Δ Anion gap) should equal the change in serum HC03 level (ΔHC03) in metabolic acidosis

That is
**Δ Anion gap should be equal to Δ HC03**

If the Δ Anion gap is > Δ HC03

Or

Δ Anion gap / Δ HC03 is > 1

Then there is an additional metabolic alkalosis

(Since normal serum HC03 is 24 thus means the patient serum HC03 did not decrease as much as it should or was actually higher than 24 if there did not occur the increase in anion gap by the acidosis)

If the Δ Anion gap is < Δ HC03

Or Δ Anion gap / Δ HC03 is < 1

Then there is an additional non -anion gap metabolic acidosis (NAGMA)

*(Thus the NAGMA has actually reduced the HC03 level below 24 to begin with, before the anion gap metabolic acidosis started to decrease the HC03 further)*

## CASE PRACTICE

### C-1

A 65 yr old female patient with pneumonia, now in septic shock with PH 7.12, PCO2 41, Na 137 chloride 96 HCO3 17   Albumin 1.9 lactate 4.1

Using what we have learnt so far-

A **First**- what is the primary acid base disorder-

metabolic acidosis- low PH, low HCO3

B **Second**- is he well compensated? – Now we bring in the winter formula

$PCO2 = 1.5 \times (17) + 8 = 25.5 + 8 = 33.5$

Since the calculated PCO2 (33.5) is more than 2 below the actual (provided pc02 of 41) then the patient is also in respiratory acidosis

So she has both a primary metabolic acidosis and a respiratory acidosis.

**C** Is there a third acid base disorder?

### What is the Anion gap

$AG = Na - (HCO3 + CL) = 137 - (96 + 17) = 137 - 113 = 24$

So calculated Anon gap = 24, however remember the serum albumin is low at 1.9

$\Delta$ Albumin = 4-1.9 = 2.1

So the anion gap will increase by 2.1 multiply by 3.5

Therefore actual anion gap = $24 + (2.1 \times 3.5) = 24 + 7.35 = 31.5$

Since normal anion gap is 12, but the patient anion gap is more than 12, that means it is a primary Anion gap metabolic acidosis

So we know that she has primary metabolic acidosis (which has just be shown to be an anion gap type) and a respiratory acidosis

To see if a third acid base disorder is also there – like a non –anion gap metabolic acidosis or a metabolic alkalosis

So we need the Δ anion gap and Δ HCO3

Δ AG = 31.5 – 12 = 19.5

Δ HCO3 - 24 - 17 = 7

Since the Δ AG is > Δ HCO3 then the patient has an additional metabolic acidosis which has to be a Non anion gap metabolic acidosis

So the patient has an Anion gap metabolic acidosis + Respiratory acidosis + Non anion gap metabolic acidosis - **Triple acid base disorder**

## Summary

Simply put–

When there is an anion gap metabolic acidosis, add the Δ anion gap to the provided serum HCO3. If the value is greater than 24 then there is a metabolic alkalosis and if the value is less than 24 then there is a metabolic acidosis.

*That is*
*For any patient in metabolic acidosis just do*

1   Na- (HCO3 + CL + 12) = if positive this equals Δ AG (that means it is also anion gap MA)
Then

*2   Add value of Δ AG to HCO3 (again) value, if more than 24 additional met alkalosis if less than 24 additional met acidosis. (Because the rules are not set in stones values within 1 of 24 e.g. 23-25 is considered normal)*

Then go ahead and apply winter formula to check for the adequacy of respiratory compensation (third disorder)

In addition, for this example since the anion gap is 19 above normal, the lactate elevation is not totally responsible for all the acidosis since the Δ anion gap more than the lactate level of 4 ( remember lactate 1:1 relationship with anion gap), that means another form of acidosis is contributing the remaining anion gap of 15 (19-4.1)

*Note during calculation for acid base disorders;*
*__1__ Always use the serum bicarbonate level measured in the blood and not in the arterial blood gas (which is actually a calculation from the PCo2 and only an estimate).*
*__2__ The actual measured serum sodium should be use not the corrected sodium for the glucose level*

## V

## CALCULATION OF BICARBONATE DEFICIT

This is the amount of HC03 needed to replace to correct a metabolic acidosis state

HCO3 deficit  =   HCO3 space  x   HCO3 deficit per liter

Bicarbonate space  =   [0.4 + (2.6 ÷ [HCO3])] x body weight (in kg)

*The space is adjusted for buffering in bone and extracellular buffers but you don't need any of the above formula*

### Hints

When serum HCO3 is between 5-10 meq/dl

Bicarbonate deficit = 70% x weight x change in HC03

Change in hc03 = 24 or value desired minus serum value

When serum HC03 <5meq/dl then

Bicarbonate deficit = 100% x weight x change in HC03

## Case Practice

### D-1

In an ICU patient in metabolic acidosis whose weight is 100kg and a serum HC03 of 8 meq, amount needed to raise it to 24 will be

Bicarbonate deficit = 70%  x   100 x (24-8)

$$= 0.7 \times 100 \times 16$$

$$= 1120 \text{ meq}$$

Since 1 ampoule of bicarbonate is 50meq, this correction will require 7.5 L (1120/150) of D5W with 3 amps of HC03 IV fluid or 15 L of half normal saline with 1 ½ amps of HC03.

However if the serum HC03 was 4meq/dl then the formula will be

Bicarbonate deficit = 100% x 100 x (24-4)

$$= 1 \times 100 \times 20$$

$$= 2000 \text{meq}$$

This will require 13.3L of D5W with 3 amps of HC03 IVF.

In the board exam questions , the values in the options are usually in multiple of tens like 65, 650, 6500, 3500 so even if the exact calculated number is not right, you can choose the closest to your value in the options

Know about D-lactic acidosis, Ativan gtt (propylene glycol) and **Pyroglutamic acidosis** in sepsis, acetaminophen and fluoxacillin use

## VI

### Urine Anion Gap

Use to determine GI loss or distal RTA as a cause of non anion gap metabolic acidosis since both conditions will have low K and serum HCO3.

In a steady state

$$\text{Urine cations} = \text{Urine anions}$$

$$(Na + K) + NH_4^+ = Cl$$

However ammonium is not readily measured. Thus to obtain urine $NH_4^+$ from the above formula

Urine CL $- (Na + K) =$ Urine $NH_4^+$

Since the normal urine anion gap is a reciprocal of the urine ammonium level

Urine AG = Measured cations - measured anions

Urine AG $= (Na + K) - CL$

In intact kidney function with normal ammoniagenesis, urine ammonium level should be > 10 thus making the urine anion gap negative (when renal excretion of ammonium is intact as in GI loss of HCO3).

But when ammonium generation and excretion by the kidney is impaired as in distal RTA, the urine anion gap becomes positive

$$\text{Urine AG} = Na + K - (CL) \quad \text{Negative in GI}$$

That is urine chloride > sum of urine sodium and potassium (because NH4 is also there to make up for the difference in cations)

Urine AG = Na + K − CL     Positive value in RTA

Urine chloride ≤ sum of urine sodium and potassium (because little or no $NH_4^+$ is excreted in the urine.

**Remember** - Do not bother to use urine anion gap in only anion gap metabolic acidosis.
It is only helpful in non anion gap metabolic acidosis

## VII

## Fractional excretion of HC03

$$FEHCO3 = \frac{\text{Urine HC03/ Serum HC03}}{\text{Urine Creatinine / Serum Creatinine}}$$

Or simply put

$$Fe\ HC03 = \frac{\text{Urine HC03} \times \text{serum Creatinine}}{\text{Serum HC03} \times \text{Urine Creatinine}}$$

**FeHC03 (%)** = $\frac{\textbf{Urine Hc03} \times \textbf{Scr}}{\textbf{Serum Hc03} \times \textbf{urine Creatinine}} \times \textbf{100}$

Useful in identifying types of Renal tubular acidosis (RTA)

**FeHC03** above 5% suggest increase renal excretion of bicarbonate as in RTA.


### Use in Types of RTA

Type 1 RTA – FeHC03 >5%
Type 2 RTA - Variable but usually >10% when serum HC03 > 18
Type 4 RTA - Variable

## VIII

### Normal Compensation for Other Acid Base Disorders

### Metabolic Alkalosis

Expected PCO2 should be

$$PCO2 = 40 + 0.7 \times \Delta HCO3$$

**Simply put**

$$\Delta PCO2 = 0.7 \times \Delta HCO3$$

*Where*

*Δ HCO3 = Serum HCO3 - 24*

*Δ PCO2 = Measured PCO2 - 40*

### In metabolic alkalosis

**Urine Chloride < 10** suggests GI loss (chloride responsive MA)

**Urine chloride > 10** suggests Renal mediated hyperaldosteronism (Non chloride responsive).

That is the kidney is dumping too much chloride and reabsorbing HCO3 excessively usually under the influence of aldosterone.
When associated with Na+ reabsoprtion, patient will have associated HTN.

### Case Practice

### E-1

77 yr old male with hypertension, remote history of tobacco use admitted now for pneumonia, patient clinically appears dehydrated, lab studies shows

Sodium       136
Chloride      97
Bicarbonate  34
Albumin      3.7
**Potassium  4.1**
**Calcium    9.0**

Arterial Blood gas shows

pH     7.39
PCO2    60
PO2     92
HCO3    22

In this case the primary disorder is Alkalosis

And since there is also elevated serum bicarbonate level, then the disorder is *Primary Metabolic alkalosis*

*To assess for respiratory compensation, we need to utilize respiratory changes for metabolic alkalosis.*

**Δ PCO2 = 0.7 x ΔHCO3**

ΔPCO2 = 0.7 x 34-24

$\quad$ = 0.7 x 10

**= 7**

Thus the PCO2 should be 7 ± 2 of the normal usual of 45.
Since the patient PCO2 is actually higher than the expected 50-54, then the patient had an additional respiratory acidosis which is likely chronic respiratory acidosis

**Renal compensation formula in Primary Respiratory disorders**

**Respiratory Acidosis**

*Acute respiratory acidosis – 1*

For every 10mmhg increase in PCO2 above 40mmhg, Serum HC03 increase by 1 above 24

That is

$\Delta HC03 = \Delta PC02 / 10$

*Chronic Respiratory acidosis - 4*

For every 10mmhg increase in PC02 above 40mmhg, serum HC03 increase by 4 above 24.

That is

$$\frac{\Delta HC03}{4} = \frac{\Delta PC02}{10}$$

**There fore**

$\Delta HC03 = \Delta PC02 / 2.5$

**Respiratory Alkalosis**

*Acute respiratory alkalosis  2*

For every 10mmhg decrease in PCO2 below 40mmhg, serum HC03 decrease by 2 below 24

$$\frac{\Delta HC03}{2} = \frac{\Delta PC02}{10}$$

**Therefore**

$\Delta HCO3 = \Delta PCO2 / 5$

### *Chronic respiratory alkalosis  5*

For every 10mmg decrease in PCO2 below 40mmhg, serum HC03 decrease by 5

That is

$$\frac{\Delta HCO3}{5} = \frac{\Delta PCO2}{10}$$

Therefore

**$\Delta HCO3 = \Delta PCO2 / 2$**


## Mnemonic to remember renal compensation changes in respiratory disorders

**1425**  (Turns out nothing too important happened in history that year)

For every 10mmg change in PC02

| | |
|---|---|
| Acute resp acidosis | - **1** |
| Chronic resp acidosis | - **4** |
| Acute resp alkalosis | - **2** |
| Chronic resp alkalosis | - **5** |

This is the normal renal response.

if the value does not correlate then there is another disorder present.

## Case Practice

### F-1

A 72-year-old morbidly obese male with past medical history of Hypertension and chronic tobacco is admitted for cough with sputum. Chest x-ray show right lobe pneumonia. Patient labs shows

| | | | |
|---|---|---|---|
| Serum Na | 134 | Serum Potassium | 5.1 |
| Serum Cl | 98 | Serum HC03 | 17.6 |
| Serum BUN | 40 | Creatinine | 3.6 |
| Serum Albumin | 3.7 | Lactate | 5.6 |
| Glucose | 514 | | |
| Ketones | trace | | |

Arterial blood Gas

| | |
|---|---|
| pH | 7.29 |
| pCO2 | 45 |
| pO2 | 75 |
| HC03 | 22.5 |

The acid base disorder here is

Step 1

The low HC03 and pH <7.4-  *suggest presence of metabolic acidosis*

Step 2

Calculate anion gap

```
AG= Na – (HC03 + CL)
   = 134- (98 + 17.6)
   = 134- 116
   = 18
```

**ΔAG = 18 – 12= 6**   s*uggest presence of anion gap metabolic acidosis*

### ΔAG + HC03 = 6 + 17.6 = 23.6

***Therefore change in serum bicarbonate was essentially due to the anion gap metabolic acidosis (no presence of additional non anion gap metabolic acidosis or metabolic alkalosis)***

Step 3

Use winters formula to identify the adequacy of respiratory compensation

1.5 x HCO3 + 8   should be within PCO2 ± 2

1.5 x 17.6 + 8 = 3

Since measured PCO2 of 45 is higher than the expected PCO2 of 35, this will suggest an additional presence *of respiratory acidosis*

**So there is an anion gap metabolic acidosis and respiratory acidosis**


**F- 2**

A 25 yr old male comes in with respiratory distress with following labs
PH 7.43   PCO2   21   HCO3 22

What is the disorder?

A   Acute respiratory alkalosis
B   Chronic respiratory acidosis
C   Combined acute respiratory alkalosis and metabolic acidosis
D   Chronic respiratory alkalosis

So here

First - we identify a primary respiratory alkalosis (low HCO3, low PCO2, high PH)

Then
$$\Delta PCO2 \ = 40-21\ = 19$$

And

$$\Delta HCO3\ = 24-22\ =\ 2$$

**That means for every 10mmhg increase in PCO2, the serum HC03 increase by almost 2**

This is consistent with acute respiratory alkalosis with normal renal compensation

Option B is incorrect because the serum HC03 should have been greater than 24
Option C is incorrect because the serum HC03 should have been lower than 22
Option is incorrect because the decrease in serum HC03 should have been by 8

## IX

### Metabolic Acidosis in chronic Kidney disease

Identify relationship between serum HC03 with elevation in Creatinine in CKD

**HC03 = 24- 0.6 (Creatinine level)**
<sub>Widmer et al ( Arch Intern Med 1979)</sub>

So for a patient with DM, HTN, CKD stage 3 with a routine clinic visit baseline Creatinine of 3.1 and a serum HC03 of 18, normal anion gap and well compensated respiratory values

You may want to check for other causes of additional metabolic acidosis such as type IV RTA since the expected HC03 should have been

Expected HC03 = 24- 0.6 (3.1)

= 24 − 1.86

= 22.14

**Chapter 2**

**BODY COMPARTMENTS VOLUMES**

## BODY FLUID COMPARTMENTS CALCULATIONS

**Total Body Water** = k x body weight ( kg)

Where    k    - 0.6 ( 60%) in Male < 55 years
- 0.55 in female <55 years
- 0.5 in elderly > 55

**Total body water = ECF water + ICF water**

ECF - extracellular water
ICF- intracellular water

Usually

ICF water = 2/3 of Total body water
ECF water = 1/3 of Total body water

And

**Plasma water = 1/4 ECF water**

Therefore

**Total body water = ECF water + ICF water**
    TBW                (1/3 TBW)            (2/3 TBW)

Plasma water    =   ¼ ECF water

                 =   ¼ x 1/3 Total body water

So

Plasma Water = 1/12 Total body water

Blood Volume = $\dfrac{\text{Plasma water}}{1-\text{HCT}}$

Remember plasma water is not same as Total Body water (which is 60% of body weight)

Knowing the volume compartments is very important in calculating electrolytes changes especially sodium and potassium in various compartments in cases of hyponatremia or hypernatremia

Plasma water concentration of any electrolytes is what is measured as serum values in routine labs

Case Practice

2A- 1

A 52 year old 100kg man with hematocrit of 36%, the plasma water will be

Total body water = $\dfrac{60}{100} \times 100 = 60L$

Therefore

Plasma water = 1/12 of 60L

= 5 L

**Blood Volume = $\dfrac{\text{Plasma water}}{1- \text{HCT}}$**

= $\dfrac{5}{1- 0.36}$

= 5 / 0.64

= 7.8 L

In this patient the ECF volume would have been 1/3 x 60 = 20L and the ICF 2/3 x 60 = 40L

2A-2

75 year old female with weight of 70 kg is seen in the office, what is the estimated plasma volume

Total body water = 55% x weight

= 0.55 x 70

= 38.5 L

Plasma volume = 1/12 x TBW

= 1/12 x 38.5

= 3.2 L

**Chapter 3**

**1- SODIUM AND WATER BALANCE**

**2 -ELECTROYLTES EXCRETION FRACTIONS**

**SODIUM AND WATER BALANCE**

**I**

Tonicity and Osmolality

Serum Osmolality =

$$2\, Na\, (mmols) + Glucose\, (mols) + Urea\, (mols)$$

Which is

$$Serum\ osmolality = 2\, Na\,(meq) + \frac{Glucose\,(mg)}{18} + \frac{Urea\,(mg)}{2.8}$$

Thus

A stable 54 yr old male with serum sodium of 138meq/l and weight of 70 kg

Total body water volume (TBW) = 0.6 x weight = 0.6 x 70

= 42 L

Total body sodium level = 42 x 138

= 5796 meq

Intracellular fluid volume = 2/3 x TBW = 2/3 x 42

= 28 L

Total intracellular sodium = 28 x 138

= 3864 meq

Extracellular fluid volume   = TBW − ICF = 14 L

　　　　　　　　　　　　　Or

　　　　　　　　　　　　= 1/3 TBW   = 14 L

Total Extracellular sodium   = TBWna − ICF na = 1932 meq

　　　　　　　　　　　　　Or

　　　　　　　　　　　　= 1/3 × TBW na   = 1932 meq

　　　　　　　　　　　　　Or

　　　　　　　　　　　　= 138 × 14   = 1932 meq

In a 100kg patient with a total body water of 60L and plasma water of 5 L, if his serum Na is 140meq/L then his total sodium in the plasma water will be 5× 140meq/L = 700meq

Since plasma water   = ¼ ECF water

Total ECF water sodium = 4 × 700

　　　　　　　　　　= 2800 meq

Then

Total body water sodium = 3 × 2800 = 8400 meq

Thus in this patient total ECF sodium is 2800meq, his ICF is 5600meq (8400-2800) and his total body sodium is 8400 meq.

From knowing the ICF total volume and total sodium amount, you can calculate the concentration of sodium in the ICF which will be (5600/40) = 140meq/L (same as the ECF serum concentration)

However it is important to know that the ICF osmolality does not change rapidly with correction of acute Hyponatremia or Hypernatremia, instead the ICF volume can contract or expand to accommodate the decrease or increase in ECF and total body sodium concentration

In rapid correction of Hyponatremia the rapid shift in osmolality gradient between the ICF and the ECF will result in fluid loss from the ICF and contraction of the ICF leading demyelination in the nervous system and clinical central pontine demyelination syndrome ( CPM)

In rapid correction of Hypernatremia the reverse will occur, the ICF *volume will expand causing a cerebral edema*

Case Practice

Case 2B-1

A 45 year old healthy male is seen for routine follow up visit. His weight is 90 kg.

His Laboratory values shows

| | |
|---|---|
| Na | 138 |
| Chloride | 101 |
| Potassium | 3.9 |
| Glucose | 140 |
| Albumin | 3.6 |
| Total protein | 8.0 |
| Bicarbonate (HC03) | 23 |
| BUN | 34 |
| Creatinine | 1.1 |

What is approximate total body sodium level

A  7450 meq

B  8900 meq

C  4968 meq

D  2484 meq

Total body water = 0.6 × 90
= 54 L

Total body Sodium = 54 × 138

= 7452 meq

2B-2

In a 100kg patient with acute decrease in serum Na level to 128meq/l who is corrected rapidly to 140meq/l in 3-4 hours, what happens to the ECF and ICF volumes

TBW patient is 60L   (60 % x weight)

Total body water sodium is = TBW x serum sodium

$$= 60 \times 128$$
$$= 9216 \text{ meq}$$

ICF water sodium =   2/3 x 92160= 6144meq

ECF sodium      = 1/3   x9216 =   3072 meq

## II

## Hyponatremia Correction

2 formulas

### I Classical formula

Sodium amount needed (deficit) = $\Delta$ Na x TBW

$\Delta$Na = change in sodium from 140

That is
= 140- new sodium level

Since Total body water (TBW) = 0.6 x weight in kg   for men
= 0.5 x weight in kg   for women or age> 65

Therefore

Sodium deficit =   weight x 0.6 x change in sodium

### II Adrogue and Madias Formula

In hypernatremia or hyponatremia, each liter of any intravenous solution used to correct the condition will raise or decrease the sodium level by

$$= \frac{(\text{Solution Sodium} + \text{solution potassium}) - \text{Serum sodium}}{\text{TBW} + 1}$$

Case Practice

2C-1

A 70 year 70 kg old male with sodium of 123, what is the sodium deficit

**Using the Classic formula**

Sodium deficit = TBW x ΔNa
= 70 x 0.5 x (140-123)
= 35 x 17
= 595 meq

Since 1L of NS (or 0.9% saline) contain 154meq of sodium per L of water. That means 595/154 = 3.8L of NS will be needed to address the deficit

Or

Since hypertonic saline (3%) contain 514meq of sodium in 1L, it will require 595/514= 1.15 L of hypertonic saline to correct the deficit.

In ideal clinical setting, correction of deficit requires calculating sodium deficit and adding the ongoing total sodium loss in urine or GI to the amount.

2C-2

Using Madias formula

A patient with hyponatremia serum sodium 123, weight 70 kg and choice of NS is being used.

Each Liter of NS will raise the serum sodium by

$$= \frac{154 - 123}{(70 \times 0.5) + 1}$$

$$= \frac{31}{35 + 1}$$

= 31/ 36

= 0.86

Replacement solution Na - 154

Replacement solution k - 0

TBW = 50% of weight

is infusion of 1L of NS will raise the serum sodium by 0.8meq, so to raise it to you will need approximately 0.8 x 17 = 14.6L of NS

contrast with the 3.8L needed to correct the deficit as shown with the first ula.
y experience, the Madias formula is not very reliable and it is only useful when patient body weight is small.

## Water Clearance Calculation

to calculate the amount of free water in any volume of urine.

formulas available:

Free water clearance Calculation

water clearance =

$$\left(1 - \frac{\text{Urine osmolality}}{\text{Plasma osmolality}}\right) \times \text{Urine volume}$$

very accurate, not used routinely anymore

Electrolyte free water Calculation

trolyte free water =

$$\left(1 - \frac{\text{Urine Na + K}}{\text{Plasma Na}}\right) \times \text{Urine volume}$$

e accurate and reliable

A positive electrolyte free water calculation means there is an additional volume of free water in the urine after excretion of the obligatory volume of water needed to remove the electrolytes

**It is usually a net positive free water excretion when Urine Na + K is < plasma Na**

**When urine Na + K > plasma Na, calculation will be negative**, suggesting instead of water excretion there is actually excess electrolyte free water absorption from the urine

Hints
- Helpful to identify SIADH (where calculation will give a negative value)

-Calculating the electrolyte free water can also be used to estimate the volume of water restriction needed

**For Example:**
A patient with urine Na 79   K 51, plasma Na 121, and urine volume of 2000mls/day, what is the maximum free water restriction needed

Urine Na + k= 79 + 51= 130

$$FEW = \left(1 - \frac{130}{121}\right) \times 2000$$

$$= (1 - 1.074) \times 2000$$

$$= -0.074 \times 2000$$

$$= \mathbf{-148 mls}$$

That means in this patient with hyponatremia, there is complete absence of electrolyte free water excretion rather more free water is being reabsoprtion from the tubules.
The usual urine sodium to water balance is being exceeded by a negative of 148 mls of water from the urine further making the hyponatremia worse

So free water restriction alone will not improve this hyponatremia.

Correcting this hyponatremia will involve reducing renal secretion of sodium and reducing tubular reabsorption of water by blocking the action of ADH.

However if in the example urine Na was 44 and K of 31

Then

FEW  $= (1- 44 + 31/ 121) \times V$

$= (1- 75 / 121) \times 2000$

$= (1- 0.6) \times 2000$

$= 0.4 \times 2000$

$= 800mls$

Since there is a positive free water excretion, restricting free water intake to less than 800cc alone will improve the hyponatremia.

Clinically very difficult to restrict water to <1000cc per day . Remember coffee, soup, soda all have over 90% water

Case Practice

2D-1

56 yr old female with seizure disorder, HTN, depression, on Sertraline admitted for dizziness, headaches and recurrent falls at home

Vitals   BP 134 / 78   Pulse 65   Resp rate 16   Temp 98.9 F   Weight 60kg

Admission labs

| | |
|---|---|
| Na | 124 |
| Chloride | 90 |
| Potassium | 3.6 |

Glucose 89

Albumin 3.6

Total protein 8.0

Bicarbonate (HC03) 22

BUN 6

Creatinine 0.5

Urine studies

PH 7.0

Na 96

Potassium 40

Chloride 56

Osmolality 890mosm/kg

24hr urine volume – 1800mls

What is the sodium deficit?

Sodium deficit = TBW x $\Delta$ Na

= (60 x 0.55) x (140-124)

= 528 mEQ

2D-2

In the above patient, will free water restriction alone correct the hyponatremia?

Electrolyte free water =

$$\left(1 - \frac{\text{Urine Na} + \text{K}}{\text{Plasma Na}}\right) \times \text{Urine volume}$$

= (1 - 96 + 40 / 124) × 1800

= (1 - 136/124) × 1800

= (1 - 1.09) × 1800

= - 0.09 × 1800

= - 162 mls

This suggest patient is secreting no electrolyte free water but rather absorbing more free water than needed ( given the negative sign) which would further worsen the hyponatremia.

**Thus free water restriction alone will not correct the hyponatremia**


2D-2

35 year old female with history of Diabetes mellitus admitted for cellulites

Vital  BP 105/68  Pulse 89  Temp 99.9  RR 18  no orthostatic

Weight 76kg

| Na | 128 | Chloride | 89 |
|---|---|---|---|
| Potassium | 4.5 | Glucose | 580 |

Albumin    3.6              Total protein    8.0

Bicarbonate (HC03)   20.4

BUN        10               Creatinine       0.6

Serum osmolality -   300 mosm/kg

Urine studies

PH         6.8              Na       67

Potassium  22               Chloride 43

Osmolality     810 mosm/kg    24hr urine volume – 3000mls

What is the best measure to correcting her serum sodium?

A  Lactate Ringers Solution

B  Normal saline

C  Insulin

D  ½ NS at 100cc/hr

Correct answer is C

Though hyponatremia but given normal osmolality, there is no urgent need for sodium replacement

## Adjust serum sodium for glucose

Each 100mg increase in serum glucose above 100, serum sodium increase by average 1.6

Actual Serum sodium =

$$\text{Measured serum Na} + \frac{(\text{Glucose} - 100)}{100} \times 1.6$$

$$= 120 + (580-100)/100 \times 1.6$$

= 128 + 480/100 x 1.6 = 128 + 4.8 x 1.6

= 128 + 7.68

= 135 meq/dl

## Hypernatremia

Remember in hypernatremia it is not sodium excess but rather water deficit in relation to sodium loss. Unlike in hyponatremia where there is actual sodium loss

I

## Correction of Hypernatremia

Classic formula

$$\text{Water deficit (L)} = \frac{\text{Serum Na} - 140}{140} \times \text{TBW}$$

Or

$$\text{Water deficit} = \text{TBW} \times \left(1 - \frac{\text{Desired Na}}{\text{Serum Na}}\right)$$

## Case Practice

2E-1

A 86 yr old female with Dementia, Hypertension, Nursing home resident admitted for new lethargy and altered mental status Current weight of 45kg

| | | | |
|---|---|---|---|
| Na | 163 | Chloride | 120 |
| Potassium | 3.5 | Glucose | 89 |
| Albumin | 3.6 | Total protein | 8.0 |
| Bicarbonate (HC03) | 28 | BUN | 86 |
| Creatinine | 2.5 | | |

ABG studies

| | | | |
|---|---|---|---|
| PH | 7.40 | PC02 | 43 |
| P02 | 70 | Hc03 | 30 |

Urine studies

| | | | |
|---|---|---|---|
| PH | 7.0 | Na | 40 |
| Potassium | 30 | Chloride | 8 |
| Osmolality | 890mosm/kg | Specific gravity | 1.040 |

**Calculate the volume of free water needed to correct the hypernatremia**

Total body water in this patient

= 45 x 0.5

= 22.5 L

0.5 of weight is being used here since elderly and female

Free water deficit

$$= \frac{163 - 140}{140} \times \text{Total body water}$$

= 23/140 x 22.5

= 3.6 L

Total free water deficit in this patient is 3.6 L.


2E-2

56 yr old male with Hypertension, Diabetes Mellitus admitted for pneumonia with cellulites. He was treated with Vancomycin and developed increase in Creatinine to 5.3 mg/dl. Creatinine subsequently trended down to 2.0 on hospital #8

Laboratory values on day #9 shows

| | | | |
|---|---|---|---|
| Na | 151 | Chloride | 101 |

Potassium        3.9         Glucose                  140

Albumin        3.6        Total protein               8.0

Bicarbonate (HCO3)       23

BUN          43        Creatinine                    1.6

Urine studies

Urine volume     3.5 L

Osmolality      420mosm/kg   Specific gravity    1.015

Weight today 84 kg

What is the free water deficit?

Total body water = 84 x 0.6

$$= 50.4 \text{ L}$$

Free water deficit

$$= \frac{151 - 140}{140} \times \text{Total body water}$$

$$= 11/140 \times 50.4$$

$$= 3.96 \text{ L}$$

Total free water deficit in this patient is 3.9 L.

## II

## Hypernatremia associated with Polyuria

*Helpful hints*

**Polyuria**   Urine volume > 3L

When urine osmolality > 800mosm/kg
- insensible water loss
- GI water loss
- Sodium intake

When Urine osmolality < 800mosm/kg

Indicate renal loss
- DI
- Osmotic diuresis-urea, glucose mannitol induced

**ELECTROYLTES EXCRETION FRACTIONS**

## Fractional Excretion of Electrolytes

-Based largely on any electrolyte excretion in relation to renal excretion of Creatinine

## Fractional excretion of Sodium

$$FeNa (\%) = \frac{\text{Urine Na} \times \text{Scr}}{\text{Serum Na} \times \text{Ucr}} \times 100$$

Scr = serum Creatinine
Ucr = urine Creatinine

Use- Helpful in identifying causes of pre-renal causes of acute renal failure

where

FeNa < 1% - pre-renal acute renal failure
FeNa > 2% - other causes

Between 1-2% is borderline

## Fractional excretion of UREA

Fractional Excretion of Urea (FEUrea)

= $(Serum_{Cr} * U_{Urea}) / (Serum_{Urea} \times U_{Cr})$ %

$$= \frac{\text{Urine Urea} \times \text{Serum cr}}{\text{Serum Urea} \times \text{Urine cr}} \times 100$$

Scr = Serum Creatinine
Ucr = urine Creatinine

Use - Helpful in differentiating Acute renal failure like FeNa, but best in cases of diuretics administration

A **fractional excretion of urea** of < 35% is suggestive of pre-renal azotemia

A fractional excretion of >50% is more suggestive of intrinsic renal injury

**Fractional Excretion of Bicarbonate**

$$FEHCO_3 = \frac{Urine\ HCO_3 / Serum\ HCO_3}{Urine\ Creatinine / Serum\ Creatinine} \times 100$$

Or simply put

$$Fe\ HCO_3 = \frac{Urine\ HCO_3 \times serum\ Creatinine}{Serum\ HCO_3 \times Urine\ Creatinine} \times 100$$

$$\mathbf{FeHCO_3\ (\%) = \frac{Urine\ HcO_3 \times Scr}{Serum\ HcO_3 \times urine\ Creatinine} \times 100}$$

Use- In identifying types of Renal tubular acidosis (RTA)

**FeHCO3** above 5% suggest increase renal excretion of bicarbonate as in Type I RTA.

**Use in Types of RTA**

Type 1 RTA – FeHCO3 >5%
Type 2 RTA - Variable but usually >10% when serum HCO3 > 18
Type 4 RTA - Variable

**Fractional excretion of Potassium**

Since potassium excretion is largely dependent on the reabsorption of sodium and water and the transtubular gradient of water across the tubular wall

The fractional excretion of potassium is calculated as the **Transtubular Potassium Gradient (TTKG)**

$$TTKG = \frac{Urine\ K\ /\ Serum\ K}{Urine\ Osm\ /\ Serum\ Osm}$$

Where urine K – urine potassium concentration
Serum K - serum potassium level
Urine Osm - urine osmolality
Serum Osm = serum osmolality

Therefore

$$TTKG = \frac{Urine\ k\ \times\ serum\ Osm}{Serum\ K\ \times\ urine\ Osm}$$

-Use to differentiate renal cause of potassium wasting or failure of excretion in both hyperkalemia and hypokalemia

**However the TTKG only effective when urine sodium is > 25**

**TTKG interpretation**

**In Hyperkalemia** when

| | |
|---|---|
| TTKG <3 | - Renal etiology from hypoaldosteronism |
| TTKG 3-7 | - Borderline for renal etiology |
| TTKG > 7 | - Hyperkalemia not related to renal etiology |

**In Hypokalemia**

TTKG > 7        - Renal etiology- likely hyperaldosetronism

TTKG 3-7      - Borderline for renal cause

TTKG <3        - Not related to renal, likely GI or poor intake.

Remember the best way to identify renal cause of hypokalemia or hyperkalemia is by 24 hr urine for potassium

24 hr urine potassium > 30meq in hypokalemia is indicative of renal etiology and the reverse of < 30meq in hyperkalemia is also suggestive


Case Practice

**3A-1**


A 43 year old female with Diabetes Mellitus, Hypertension, on high potassium diet prescribed as a measure to help hypertension by her friends; she is admitted for weakness and muscle aches

Home meds- Amlodipine, hydrochlorothiazide, ibuprofen

| | | | |
|---|---|---|---|
| Na | 132 | Chloride | 92 |
| Potassium | 7.2 | Glucose | 140 |
| Albumin | 3.6 | Total protein | 8.0 |
| Bicarbonate (HC03) | 20 | | |
| BUN | 18 | Creatinine | 1.0 |
| Serum osmolality | | 292 mosm/kg | |
| Arterial pH | | 7.33 | |

Random Urine studies shows:

Osmolality        510mosm/kg    Specific gravity    1.035

Urine sodium     95           Urine potassium    35

## What is the likely cause of her hyperkalemia?

A High potassium diet

B Functional Hypoaldosteronism

C Ibuprofen use

D Hyperglycemia induced

## Calculate the TTKG

$$= \frac{\text{urine K} \times \text{serum osmolality}}{\text{Serum K} \times \text{urine osmolality}}$$

$$= \frac{35 \times 292}{510 \times 7.2}$$

$= 2.7$

Since less than 3.5 insetting of hyperkalemia, likely cause of hyperkalemia is impaired renal excretion of potassium from functional or absolute deficiency in Aldosterone

**Correct answer is B**

### Fractional excretion of Uric acid

$$F_{Euric} = \frac{\text{Urine uric acid / Serum uric acid}}{\text{Urine Creatinine / Serum Creatinine}} \times 100$$

Or simply put

$$Fe\ uric = \frac{Urine\ uric\ acid \times serum\ Creatinine}{Serum\ uric\ acid \times Urine\ Creatinine} \times 100$$

Normal range is 6-10% male and 10-13 in female

Value of < 6 % suggest impaired Urate excretion as in familial Juvenile Hyperuricemic nephropathy FJHN (also called Medullary cystic kidney disease)

# Chapter 4

## KIDNEY DISEASE STATES AND ELECTROLYTES CHANGES

1- Acute renal Failure

2- Chronic kidney disease

3- Nutrition in renal failure

# 1 Acute Renal failure

- Helpful in differentiating cases of pre-renal and intrinsic renal injuries

## Fractional excretion of Sodium

$$FeNa (\%) = \frac{\text{Urine Na} \times \text{Scr}}{\text{Serum Na} \times \text{Ucr}} \times 100$$

Scr = serum Creatinine
Ucr = urine Creatinine

Helpful in identifying causes of pre-renal causes of acute renal failure, where

FeNa < 1% - pre-renal acute renal failure
FeNa > 2% - other causes

Between 1-2% is borderline

## Urine sodium

### Usually < 20 in pre-renal

However in presence of metabolic alkalosis, urine sodium can be >20 due to obligatory sodium loss with increase renal excretion bicarbonate. For example a patient with volume depletion from vomiting which developed contracture alkalosis and pre-renal Acute renal failure.

## Fractional Excretion of UREA

Fractional Excretion of Urea (FEUrea)

$$= (Serum_{Cr} * U_{Urea}) / (Serum_{Urea} \times U_{Cr}) \%$$

$$= \frac{\text{Urine Urea} \times \text{Serum cr}}{\text{Serum Urea} \times \text{Urine cr}} \times 100$$

Scr = serum Creatinine    Ucr = urine Creatinine

- Helpful in cases of diuretics use

A **fractional excretion of urea** of < 35% is suggestive of pre-renal azotemia

While fractional **excretion of urea** of >50% is suggestive of ATN

**CHRONIC KIDNEY DISEASE**

## Creatinine Clearance in chronic kidney disease

Kidney clearance- Estimated Glomular filtration rate (eGFR) calculation

3 methods:

### I  24 hr urine Creatinine Clearance

$$eGFR = \frac{Uvol \times Ucr}{Plasma\ cr}$$

Where Uvol = 24 hr urine in mls
    Ucr- Creatinine concentration in urine
    Plasma cr- plasma Creatinine

= eGFR in L/day

$$= \frac{eGFR \times 1000}{24 \times 60}$$

= eGFR in L/day x 1000/1440

= eGFR in mls/min

Remember problems with this method include-
-Unreliable 24 hr urine collection
-No accounting for increase distal tubule secretion of Creatinine with decrease in renal function
-Tubular secretion of Creatinine is affected by many drugs and agents

### II  Cockcroft Gault Formula

$$eGFR = \frac{(140 - Age) \times 72}{Weight\ in\ kg \times serum\ Creatinine} \quad \text{for men}$$

And

$$eGFR = \frac{(140 - age) \times 72 \times 0.85}{\text{Weight in kg} \times \text{serum cr}} \quad \text{for women}$$

Remember problems with this method include – unreliable result at higher GFR estimates ( > 50mls/min)

### III Modified Diet in Renal Disease –MDRD- formula

eGFR = 170 x (SCr[mg/dL])exp[-0.999] x (Age)exp[-0.176] x (BUN [mg/dL])exp[-0.170] x (Alb [g/dL])exp[+0.318] x (0.762 if female) x (1.18 if black)

Usually online

Problem with formula is same as Cockcroft Gault – both inaccurate at higher eGFR values

Case Practice

4 A- 1

70 year old female with Diabetes Mellitus, Hypertension, Obesity, chronic kidney disease present for routine follow up visit. Her weight has been stable around 90 kg with a serum creatinine of 1.9 mmol/dl. What is her calculated Creatinine clearance and kidney disease stage?

Using the Cockcroft Gault

$$\text{Creatinine clearance} = \frac{(140 - 70) \times 72 \times 0.85}{90 \times 1.9}$$

$$= \frac{70 \times 72 \times 0.85}{90 \times 1.9}$$

$$= 25 \text{ mls/min}$$

Therefore the patient is in stage IV chronic kidney disease

## Metabolic Acidosis in chronic Kidney disease

Identify relationship between serum HC03 with elevation in Creatinine in CKD

**HC03 = 24- 0.6 (Creatinine level)**

Widmer et al ( Arch Intern Med 1979)

**Nutrition in Renal failure**

**Protein prescription**

Protein replacement dosage in acute renal failure is based on Nitrogen balance calculation

**Nitrogen balance = (Protein intake /6.25) - (UUN + 4)**

Protein intake – protein intake in 24 hrs
UUN- urine urea nitrogen level in 24 hrs

Positive Nitrogen balance reflects adequate protein supplemental in acute renal failure

**Calorie prescription in Renal Failure**

Based on 24 hr Basic Energy Requirement with the Harris-Benedict equation

**Basic Energy Requirement (BER)**

= 66 + ( 13.7 x weight) + ( 5 x height) – ( 6.8 x Age) in Men

= 655 + (9.6 x weight ) + ( 1.8 x height ) – ( 4.7 x age ) in Women

Multiply value stress factor which range from 1.0 (mild stress state) to 1.4 (severe stress state)

## Normal Protein Catabolic rate

Garred Formula

Protein catabolic rate ( nPCR ) =

$[0.0504 (1 - 0.162 C_{urea}\ pre/ C_{urea}\ post)( 1 - C_{urea}\ post/ C_{urea}\ pre + \Delta BW/ 0.58 ] C_{urea}\ pre/[ ( 1 - 0.0003\ T_{HD}] + 0.17$

Where

C urea pre- urea concentration pre-HD
C urea post – urea concentration Post HD
$\Delta$ BW – change in body weight during dialysis
$T_{HD}$- duration of dialysis in hours

**Chapter 5**

**DIALYSIS RELATED FORMULAS**

I

**Peritoneal Dialysis clearance Adequacy**

$$PD\ KT/V = \frac{\text{Total dwell volume in 24 hrs} \times D/P\ \text{urea}}{\text{Urea volume of distribution in Liters}} \times 7$$

Urea volume of distribution = 0.6 x body weight (in men)
= 0.5 x body weight (women)

$$D/P\ \text{urea} = \frac{\text{Dialysate urea concentration}}{\text{Plasma urea concentration}}$$

Multiply by 7 since kt/v is average clearance in 1 week

If residual urine function (that is urine volume > 100mls /day) then add residual urine clearance

*Example* - In a PD female patient with weight 107kg total drain volume of 15.5L , dialysate urea( BUN) of 28 Creatinine 4.0 , serum BUN 49, Creatinine of 7.5. Her urine residual urine volume of 300cc with a 24hr urine clearance of 1ml/min

Then

$$PD\ KT = \frac{28/49 \times 15.5}{V} \times 7$$

V= volume of urea distribution= 0.5 x lean body weight

$$= \frac{0.57 \times 15.5 \times 7}{0.5 \times 107}$$

$$= \frac{0.57 \times 15.5 \times 7}{53.5} = \frac{8.85 \times 7}{53.5} = 0.16 \times 7 = 1.15$$

Her PD kt/v = 1.15

## II

### Residual Renal Function KT/V clearance

$$RRF\ KT/V = \frac{KT}{V}$$

First calculate the eGFR by 24 hr urine clearance in mls/min

KT = eGFR in 1 week

That is

$$KT = \frac{(eGFR\ in\ mls/min) \times 60 \times 24 \times 7}{1000 mls}$$

This gives the answer in KT in Liters

In our above patient, her residual renal function KT/V will be

$$RRF\ KT/V = \frac{1 \times 60 \times 24 \times 7}{53.5 \times 1000} = 0.18$$

So her total KT/V (sum of both PD kt/v and residual kidney kt/v) will be

$$1.15 + 0.18 = 1.33$$

However you need to adjust for BSA, in this patient her BSA is 2.08, to convert to standard 1.73 m2, her adjusted KT/V will be lower by 1.3 x 1.73/2.08

## III

### Hemodialysis Clearance Adequacy

- Usually done online

### *Daugirdas formula*

KT/V = -in [ ( Bun post/BUN pre) − ( 0.008 x hours)] +(( 4-(3.5 x Bun post/Bun pre)] x UF volume /weight Post)

That is

Kt/V = -ln (R - 0.03) + [(4 - 3.5R) x (UF ÷ W)]

Where R = Bun Post/ Bun Pre

You can always add the RRF KT/V to the HD online Daugirdas formula derived KT/V for hemodialysis patients

Case Practice

5A-1

A 21 yr old male patient with polycystic kidney disease and ESRD on hemodialysis has a 24hr urine Creatinine clearance of 8mls/min, his weight is 82kg. His online derived KT/V is 1.25

Then

Residual Renal Function ( RRF) KT =

$$\text{RRF KT} = \frac{8 \times 60 \times 24 \times 7}{1000} = 80.4$$

Volume (V) = 60% x weight

$$= 0.6 \times 82 = 49 \text{ L}$$

Then

RRF KT/V = 80/49 = 1.6

Total KT/V = HD kt/v + RRF kt/v = 1.25 + 1.6

= 2.85

5A-2

A 27 yr old male with dilated Cardiomyopathy on dialysis for Cardiorenal syndrome and persistent fluid overload, calculated dialysis KT/V is 1.09. His 24 hr urine clearance is 18 mls/min, with estimated dry weight of 210 lbs

$$\text{RRF KT} = \frac{18 \times 60 \times 24 \times 7}{1000}$$

$$V = 60\% \text{ weight} = \frac{60}{100} \times \frac{210}{2.2} = 57 \text{ L}$$

Residual renal function KT/V= 3.17

## Recirculation Calculation during hemodialysis

$$\text{Recirculation rate } (R\%) = \frac{(C_{equi} - C_{art})}{(C_{equi} - C_{ven})} \times 100$$

**Where**

$C_{equi}$ - concentration of either urea or creatinine 2 mins after reducing pump speed
$C_{art}$ - Arterial blood concentration of either urea or creatinine
$C_{ven}$ - Venous blood concentration of either urea or creatinine

**Result express as %**


## IV

## Continuous Renal Replacement Therapy (CRRT) Dose of therapy

**Dialysate flow delivered dose of 25mls/kg/hr have same outcome in terms of mortality and morbidity with dose of >35mls/kg/hr**

-Renal study and ATN study

*However, since all dose prescribed are not delivered due to many mechanical problems, in clinical practice it is safer to prescribed at doses of >25mls/kg/hr.*

## CRRT clearance calculation

### Solute clearance (K)

$$K = \frac{(QDo \times CDo - QDi \times CDi)}{Sc}$$

Where

QDi – rate of dialysate flow **in**to filter
QDo – rate of dialysate flow **out** of filter
CDi - concentration of a given solute in the dialysate flowing into the dialyzer
CDo - concentration of a given solute in the dialysate flowing out of dialyzer
Sc - concentration of the solute in the blood entering the filter which is same as serum concentration

Know the dialysate flow at the outlet will be the sum of the dialysate flow at the inlet and any UF prescribed so

$QDo = QDi + UF$

When Urea or Creatinine is the solute whose clearance is being calculated, as is usual, and since there is usually no urea or Creatinine in the dialysate, then there is not expected any urea or Creatinine in the dialysate flow into the inlet, making the concentration of urea in the inlet = 0

Therefore

$K = (QDo \times CDo - QDi \times CDi) \;/\; Sc$

$K = (QDo \times CDo - QDi \times 0) \;/\; Sc$ 　　　　　since CDi=0

$K = (QDo \times CDo - 0) \;/\; Sc$

$$K = \frac{QDo \times CDo}{Sc}$$

Thus

CRRT Solute clearance for urea or Creatinine

$$= \frac{\text{Dialysate flow in outlet} \times \text{concentration in outlet Dialysate}}{\text{Serum concentration}}$$

Remember since QDo = QDi + UF

$$K = \frac{(QDi + UF) \times CDo}{CB}$$

$$= \frac{(QDi \times CDo) + (UF \times CDo)}{Sc}$$

$$= \frac{QDi \times CDo}{Sc} + \frac{UF \times CDo}{Sc}$$

  Diffusive clearance          convective clearance

= Diffusive clearance    + convective clearance

Thus adding more UF as in CVVHDF will increase solute clearance better than CVVH where little UF can be added

Case Practice

5B-1

A 90 kg patient on vent in Surgical ICU with AKI, started on CRRT with prescribed rate of 2000mls/hr and UF 200cc/hr, if the serum Creatinine is 9mg/dl , and Dialysate Creatinine of 9mg/L. what is the Creatinine clearance ?

$$K = \frac{QDo \times CDo}{Sc}$$

Here QDo =   2000 + 200   =   2200mls
CDo = 9mg/L  = 0.9mg/dl

Then

$$K = \frac{2200 \times 0.9}{9}$$

= 220 mls/hr

= 220/60 mls/min

= 3.5 mls/min

*Which is just marginal given that 2000/90 prescription dose is just 22mls/kg/hr dose*

V

## Plasma Volume Exchange

Plasmapharesis prescription dosage

**Plasma volume (in liters) = 0.07 x weight (kg) x (1 - hematocrit)**

Another approximate method is using a volume of 40-60 mls /kg

Case Practice

5C-1

A 100kg female patient with hematocrit of 40% diagnosed with TTP, now in need of plasmapharesis, the plasma volume per procedure to ensure 70 % of plasma protein exchange will be

= 0.07 x 100 x (1-40%)

= 0.07 x 100 x 0.6

= 7x 0.6 = 4.2L

**CASE PRACTICE QUESTIONS**

**Normal ranges of values**

| | | Units |
|---|---|---|
| **Sodium** | 136 – 145 | mmol/L |
| **Potassium** | 3.5 - 5.1 | mmol/L |
| **Chloride** | 98 – 107 | mmol/L |
| **BUN, Bld** | 7 – 22 | mg/dL |
| **Creatinine** | 0.6 - 1.3 | mg/dl |
| **Glucose** | 70 - 99 | mg/dL |
| **Calcium** | **8.**5 - 10.1 | mg/dL |
| **Phosphorus** | 2.5 - 4.9 | mg/dL |
| **Albumin** | **3.**4 - 5.0 | g/dL |
| **CO2 or HC03** | 21.0 - 32.0 | mmol/L |

1

A 42 yr old female with HTN, DM, and COPD admitted for sepsis and hypotension

| | | | |
|---|---|---|---|
| Na | 140 | Chloride | 90 |
| Potassium | 3.9 | Glucose | 98 |
| Albumin | 3.9 | Total protein | 8.2 |
| Bicarbonate (HC03) | 22 | BUN | 43 |
| Creatinine | 2.5 | | |

ABG studies

| | | | |
|---|---|---|---|
| PH | 7.23 | PC02 | 50 |
| P02 | 71 | Hc03 | 23 |

What is the acid base disorder in this patient?

A Non Anion gap Metabolic Acidosis only

B Metabolic alkalosis only

C Respiratory Acidosis and Metabolic acidosis only

D Respiratory Alkalosis, Metabolic Alkalosis and Metabolic Acidosis

E Respiratory Acidosis, Metabolic Alkalosis and Metabolic Acidosis

F Anion gap Metabolic Acidosis only

2

56 yr old female with Ulcerative colitis, Diabetes Mellitus, Hypertension admitted for diarrhea

| | | | |
|---|---|---|---|
| Na | 129 | Chloride | 111 |
| Potassium | 2.8 | Glucose | 98 |
| Albumin | 3.9 | Total protein | 8.2 |
| Bicarbonate (HCO3) | 19 | BUN | 20 |
| Creatinine | 1.5 | | |

**ABG studies**

| | | | |
|---|---|---|---|
| PH | 7.34 | PCO2 | 42 |
| PO2 | 75 | HcO3 | 22 |

**Urine studies**

| | | | |
|---|---|---|---|
| PH | 6.0 | Na | 34 |
| Potassium | 16 | Chloride | 61 |
| Osmolality | 510mom/kg | | |

What is the acid base disorder in this patient?

A Non Anion gap Metabolic Acidosis only

B Metabolic alkalosis only

C Respiratory Acidosis and Metabolic acidosis only

D Respiratory Alkalosis, Metabolic Alkalosis and Metabolic Acidosis

E Respiratory Acidosis, Metabolic Alkalosis and Metabolic Acidosis

F Anion gap Metabolic Acidosis only

23 yr old female with thin built admitted for increasing weakness and diarrhea. History of regular use of weight loss supplements

| | | | |
|---|---|---|---|
| Na | 136 | Chloride | 106 |
| Potassium | 3.1 | Glucose | 101 |
| Albumin | 3.6 | Total protein | 8.0 |
| Bicarbonate ($HCO_3$) 20 | | BUN | 30 |
| | | Creatinine | 1.3 |

**ABG studies**

| | | | |
|---|---|---|---|
| PH | 7.30 | $PCO_2$ | 31 |
| $PO_2$ | 71 | $HcO_3$ | 30 |

Urine studies

| | | | |
|---|---|---|---|
| PH | 6.0 | Na | 60 |
| Potassium | 3.6 | Chloride | 5 |
| Osmolality | 510mom/kg | Specific gravity | 1.041 |

What is the acid base disorder in this patient?

A Non Anion gap Metabolic Acidosis only

B Metabolic alkalosis only

C Respiratory Acidosis and Metabolic acidosis only

D Respiratory Alkalosis, Metabolic Alkalosis and Metabolic Acidosis

E Respiratory Acidosis, Metabolic Alkalosis and Metabolic Acidosis

4

56 yr old male with COPD, Obesity, HTN, admitted for cough, sputum and SOB

| | | | |
|---|---|---|---|
| Na | 142 | Chloride | 94 |
| Potassium | 3.8 | Glucose | 101 |
| Albumin | 3.6 | Total protein | 8.0 |
| Bicarbonate (HC03) | 33 | BUN | 36 |
| Creatinine | 1.0 | | |

**ABG studies**

| | | | |
|---|---|---|---|
| PH | 7.41 | PCO2 | 56 |
| PO2 | 66 | Hc03 | 30 |

**Urine studies**

| | | | |
|---|---|---|---|
| PH | 6.0 | Na | 60 |
| Potassium | 36 | Chloride | 45 |
| Osmolality | 510mom/kg | Specific gravity | 1.041 |

What is the acid base disorder in this patient?

A Non Anion gap Metabolic Acidosis only

B Metabolic alkalosis only

C Respiratory Acidosis and Metabolic acidosis only

D Metabolic Alkalosis and Respiratory Acidosis

E Respiratory Acidosis, Metabolic Alkalosis and Metabolic Acidosis

5

A 55 yr old male with uncontrolled hypertension

| | | | | |
|---|---|---|---|---|
| Na | 142 | Chloride | | 112 |
| Potassium | 2.9 | Glucose | | 101 |
| Albumin | 3.6 | Total protein | | 8.0 |
| Bicarbonate (HC03) | 33 | BUN | | 15 |
| Creatinine | 1.0 | | | |

**ABG studies**

| | | | |
|---|---|---|---|
| pH | 7.41 | PC02 | 36 |
| P02 | 76 | Hc03 | 30 |

**Urine studies**

| | | | |
|---|---|---|---|
| PH | 6.5 | Na | 25 |
| Potassium | 41 | Chloride | 55 |
| Osmolality | 410mom/kg | Specific gravity | 1.021 |

- What is the acid base disorder in this patient?

A  Non Anion gap Metabolic Acidosis only

B  Metabolic alkalosis only

C  Respiratory Acidosis and Metabolic acidosis only

D  Respiratory Acidosis, Metabolic Alkalosis and Metabolic Acidosis

6

71 yr old female with arthritis, history of regular ibuprofen use admitted for nausea, vomiting

| | | | |
|---|---|---|---|
| Na | 135 | Chloride | 80 |
| Potassium | 3.1 | Glucose | 101 |
| Albumin | 3.6 | Total protein | 8.0 |
| Bicarbonate (HC03) | 33 | BUN | 26 |
| Creatinine | 1.5 | | |

**ABG studies**

| | | | |
|---|---|---|---|
| PH | 7.40 | PCO2 | 43 |
| PO2 | 70 | HcO3 | 30 |

**Urine studies**

| | | | |
|---|---|---|---|
| PH | 7.5 | Na | 40 |
| Potassium | 30 | Chloride | 8 |
| Osmolality | 520mom/kg | Specific gravity | 1.040 |

- What is the acid base disorder in this patient?

A Non Anion gap Metabolic Acidosis only

B Metabolic alkalosis – chloride responsive

C Respiratory Acidosis and Metabolic acidosis only

D Metabolic Alkalosis – Non Chloride responsive

7

A 86 yr old female with Dementia, Hypertension, Nursing home resident admitted for new lethargy and altered mental status
Current weight of 45kg

| | | | | |
|---|---|---|---|---|
| Na | 163 | Chloride | | 120 |
| Potassium | 3.5 | Glucose | | 89 |
| Albumin | 3.6 | Total protein | | 8.0 |
| Bicarbonate (HCO3) 28 | | BUN | | 86 |
| Creatinine | 2.5 | | | |

ABG studies

| | | | |
|---|---|---|---|
| PH | 7.40 | PCO2 | 43 |
| PO2 | 70 | HcO3 | 30 |

**Urine studies**

| | | | | |
|---|---|---|---|---|
| PH | 7.41 | Na | | 40 |
| Potassium | 30 | Chloride | | 8 |
| Osmolality | 890mosm/kg | Specific gravity | | 1.040 |

What is the calculated free water deficit?

A  5 Liters

B  3.5 Liters

C  2 Liters

D  7 Liters

8

56 yr old male with Hypertension, Diabetes Mellitus admitted for pneumonia with cellulitis. He was treated with Vancomycin and developed increase in Creatinine to 5.3 mg/dl . Creatinine subsequently trended down to 2.0 on hospital #8
Laboratory values on day #9 shows

| | | | |
|---|---|---|---|
| Na | 151 | Chloride | 101 |
| Potassium | 3.9 | Glucose | 140 |
| Albumin | 3.6 | Total protein | 8.0 |
| Bicarbonate (HCO3) | 23 | BUN | 43 |
| Creatinine | 1.6 | | |

Urine studies

Urine volume    3.5 L

Osmolality    420mosm/kg

Specific gravity    1.015

Weight today 84 kg

What is the free water deficit?

A  5 Liters

B  4 Liters

C  2 Liters

D  7 Liters

**9**

**35 yr old male with diarrhea and presumed gastroenteritis.**

**His** laboratory tests shows

Sodium 141    Chloride 109
Bicarbonate 19    Albumin 3.8
Potassium 3.4    Calcium 8.9
BUN 56    Creatinine 2.0

*Arterial blood gas analysis shows*
pH 7.36
PCO2 32
PO2 90
HCO3 33

What is the acid base disorder in this patient?

A Non Anion gap Metabolic Acidosis only

B Metabolic alkalosis – chloride responsive

C Respiratory Acidosis and Metabolic acidosis only

D Metabolic Alkalosis – Non Chloride responsive

## 10

59 yr old male with recent Nsaid use for arthritis, is admitted for heartburn, nausea and vomiting. His laboratory tests shows

Sodium 140
Chloride 112
Bicarbonate 29
Albumin 3.8
Potassium 3.0
Calcium 8.9

*Arterial blood gas analysis shows*

pH 7.42
PCO2 33
PO2 76

What is the acid base disorder in this patient?

A Non Anion gap Metabolic Acidosis only

B Metabolic alkalosis – chloride responsive

C Respiratory Acidosis and Metabolic acidosis only

D Metabolic Alkalosis – Non Chloride responsive

**11**

54 yr old male with multiple myeloma on chemotherapy, is seen in routine office visit. His laboratory tests shows

| | |
|---|---|
| Sodium | 140 |
| Chloride | 112 |
| Bicarbonate | 20 |
| Albumin | 3.8 |
| Potassium | 3.9 |
| Calcium | 8.9 |

*Arterial blood gas analysis shows*
| | |
|---|---|
| pH | 7.35 |
| PCO2 | 40 |
| HCO3 | 22 |

What is the acid base disorder in this patient?

A Non Anion gap Metabolic Acidosis only

B Metabolic alkalosis – chloride responsive

C Respiratory Acidosis and Metabolic acidosis only

D Metabolic Alkalosis – Non Chloride responsive

## 12

45 year old Caucasian female with Crohn"s disease admitted for weakness, recent onset of diarrhea. Her laboratory tests shows

| | |
|---|---|
| Sodium | 129 |
| Chloride | 102 |
| Bicarbonate | 17 |
| Albumin | 3.8 |
| **Potassium** | **3.1** |
| **Calcium** | **9.0** |

*Arterial blood gas analysis shows*

| | |
|---|---|
| pH | 7.23 |
| PCO2 | 44 |
| PO2 | 90 |
| HCO3 | 19 |

What is the acid base disorder in this patient?

A Non Anion gap Metabolic Acidosis only

B Metabolic alkalosis – chloride responsive

C Respiratory Acidosis and Metabolic acidosis

D Metabolic Alkalosis – Non Chloride responsive

## 13

58 year old female with history of seizure disorder on acetazolamide; she is seen in the Emergency room, post fall at home. Her laboratory tests shows

| | |
|---|---|
| Sodium | 134 |
| Chloride | 108 |
| Bicarbonate | 17 |
| Albumin | 3.8 |
| **Potassium** | **3.6** |
| **Calcium** | **8.5** |

*Arterial blood gas analysis shows*
pH         7.34
PCO2       30
PO2        90
HCO3       18

What is the acid base disorder in this patient?

A Non Anion gap Metabolic Acidosis only

B Metabolic alkalosis – chloride responsive

C Respiratory Acidosis and Metabolic acidosis only

D Respiratory Alkalosis and Metabolic Acidosis

## 14

A 65 year old male with history of mental retardation, schizophrenia prior lithium use admitted for weakness. His laboratory tests shows

Sodium       137
Chloride     112
Bicarbonate  20.4
Albumin      3.8
Potassium    3.7
Calcium      8.9
BUN          56
Creatinine   2.9

*Arterial blood gas analysis shows*
pH         7.27
PCO2       56
PO2        90
HCO3       56

What is the acid base disorder in this patient?

A Non Anion gap Metabolic Acidosis only

B Metabolic alkalosis – chloride responsive

C Respiratory Acidosis and Metabolic acidosis only

D Metabolic Alkalosis – Non Chloride responsive

## 17

**24 yr old female is admitted for suicide attempt with aspirin overdose. Her** laboratory tests shows

| | |
|---|---|
| Sodium | 136 |
| Chloride | 92 |
| Bicarbonate | 20 |
| Albumin | 3.8 |
| Potassium | 3.5 |
| Calcium | 8.9 |

*Arterial blood gas analysis shows*

| | |
|---|---|
| pH | 7.42 |
| $PCO_2$ | 23 |
| $PO_2$ | 90 |
| $HCO_3$ | 23 |

What is the acid base disorder in this patient?

A Non Anion gap Metabolic Acidosis only

B Metabolic alkalosis – chloride responsive

C Respiratory Acidosis and Metabolic acidosis only

D Respiratory Alkalosis

18

A 79 yr old Nursing home patient with Dementia and Hypertension, is seen in the emergency for fever and cough.

Vital signs – BP 86/45 + orthostatic  Pulse 90  Resp rate 22  Tmep 101.1

His laboratory values are

| | | | |
|---|---|---|---|
| Na | 163 | Chloride | 120 |
| Potassium | 3.5 | Glucose | 89 |
| Albumin | 3.6 | Total protein | 8.0 |
| Bicarbonate (HC03) | 28 | BUN | 86 |
| Creatinine | 2.5 | | |

ABG studies

| | | | |
|---|---|---|---|
| pH | 7.40 | PC02 | 43 |
| P02 | 70 | Hc03 | 30 |

Urine studies

| | | | |
|---|---|---|---|
| PH | 7.0 | Na | 40 |
| Potassium | 30 | Chloride | 8 |
| Osmolality | 890mosm/kg | Specific gravity | 1.040 |

What is the best measure to correcting his serum sodium?

A  Dextrose infusion

**B**  Normal saline

C  0.45% Normal Saline

D  Normal saline and furosemide

19

A 65 year old female with Depression, Hypertension is seen for a routine office visit. She has no complains. Her current medications include Sertraline, Aspirin, fish oil and metoprolol

Her laboratory values are shown below

| | | | |
|---|---|---|---|
| Na | 125 | Chloride | 89 |
| Potassium | 4.5 | Glucose | 90 |
| Albumin | 3.6 | Total protein | 8.0 |
| Bicarbonate (HC03) | 22.4 | BUN | 10 |
| Creatinine | 0.6 | | |

Serum osmolality -   272 mosm/kg

Urine studies

| | | | |
|---|---|---|---|
| PH | 6.8 | Na | 67 |
| Potassium | 22 | Chloride | 43 |
| Osmolality | 510 mosm/kg | | |

Body weight    60 kg

What is the approximate total sodium deficit?

A  514 meq

B  330 meq

C 715 meq

D 150 meq

20

A 54 yr old male with Hypertension, Diabetes Mellitus, Bipolar disorder on lithium therapy for over 10 years present in the emergency room with increasing lethargy and confusion.

His Vital signs were BP 121/78 Pulse 65 Resp 17 Temp 98.9

His physical examination was otherwise unremarkable

His Laboratory values shows

| Na | 154 | Chloride | 101 |
|---|---|---|---|
| Potassium | 3.9 | Glucose | 140 |
| Albumin | 3.6 | Total protein | 8.0 |
| Bicarbonate (HC03) | 23 | BUN | 34 |
| Creatinine | 1.1 | Serum osmolality – 295 mosm/kg | |

Urine studies

| 24 hr Urine volume | 4 L | Osmolality | 200 mosm/kg |
|---|---|---|---|
| Specific gravity | 1.015 | | |
| Weight today | 84 kg | | |

What is the approximate water deficit?

A  5 Liters

B 6 Liters

C 3 Liters

D  8 Liters

21

A 60-year-old woman with Hypertension is admitted to hospital with severe vomiting. Noted with hypotension and tachycardia 120/min.

Laboratory studies:

| Na | 138 | | Chloride | 80 |
|---|---|---|---|---|
| Potassium | 3.1 | | Glucose | 101 |
| Albumin | 3.6 | | Total protein | 8.0 |
| Bicarbonate (HC03) | | 11 | BUN | 90 |
| Creatinine | 2.8 | | | |

## ABG studies

| PH | 7.29 |
|---|---|
| PC02 | 24 |
| P02 | 70 |

What state does the patient's acid-base status indicate?

A. Non-anion gap metabolic acidosis

B. Anion gap metabolic acidosis

C. Anion gap metabolic acidosis and metabolic Alkalosis

D. Anion gap metabolic acidosis and respiratory alkalosis

## 22

A 64 year old female presented with new onset headache, weakness, fever, anemia and low platelets. She was diagnosed with thrombotic thrombocytopenic purpura and a decision to start plasmapharesis is recommended

Her data shows

Weight 76 kg

Her laboratory studies shows

| | | | |
|---|---|---|---|
| Sodium | 136 meq/L | Potassium | 5.1 meq/L |
| Chloride | 92 meq/L | HCO3 | 19 meq/L |
| Albumin | 3.4 mg/dl | Calcium | 8.4 mg/dl |
| BUN | 52 mg/dl | Creatinine | 2.1 mg/dl |
| WBC | 11,000 | Hemoglobin | 9.2 mg/dl |
| Hematocrit | 21 | Platelets | 24,000 |

What is the dose of plasma exchange volume if using 1:1 Plasma Volume?

A  4 Liters per exchange

B  3 Liters per exchange

C  2 Liters per exchange

D  8 Liters per exchange

## 23

A 82 year male with long standing hypertension is seen in his primary care office for elevated blood pressure of 161/80.

His only laboratory available is serum creatinine of 1.7. His weight today is 82 kg

What is his estimated glomerular filtrate rate?

A 29 mls/min

B 38 mls/min

C 11 mls/min

D 25 mls/min


24

An 82 year female with long standing hypertension and diabetes mellitus is seen in his primary care office for elevated blood pressure of 161/80.

His only laboratory available is serum creatinine of 1.7. Her weight today is 82 kg

What is her estimated glomerular filtrate rate?

A 29 mls/min

B 38 mls/min

C 51 mls/min

D 25 mls/min

Case Vignette for questions 25- 27

A 54 year old female with Cohn's disease, Hypertension, Congestive heart failure is admitted for increase weakness. She has an ongoing bout of watery diarrhea
Her home meds: furosemide 40 mg daily, calcium carbonate 1000mg bid, Amlodipine 10 mg daily

His Laboratory values shows

| | | | |
|---|---|---|---|
| Na | 136 | Chloride | 96 |
| Potassium | 3.9 | Glucose | 140 |
| Albumin | 3.6 | Total protein | 8.0 |
| Bicarbonate (HC03) | 19 | BUN | 56 |
| Creatinine | 2.5 | Serum osmolality | 285 mosm/kg |

Urine studies

| | | | |
|---|---|---|---|
| Specific gravity | 1.040 | Sodium | 32 |
| Potassium | 36 | Chloride | 54 |
| Urea | 140 | Creatinine | 20 |

25

What is fractional sodium excretion?

A   < 1%

B   > 2 %

C  Between 1-2 %

D < 0.5 %

26

What is fractional urea excretion?

A  <35%

B  >50%

C  35-50%

D  <10%

27

What is the likely cause of acute renal failure in the above patient?

A. Pre-renal – since FeUrea is <35% and on diuretics which can explain elevated FeNa of >2 %

B  Intrinsic renal failure – since FeNa > 2%

C  Post obstructive renal disease

D  Pre-renal – since FeNa is > 2%

28

An 80 yr old female with Dementia, nursing home patient admitted for fever and shortness of breath.

Her vital signs are    BP 145/69 Pulse 89 R 22   Temp 101.2 F

CXR done shows evidence of left lobe infiltrate

Her labs shows

| | | | |
|---|---|---|---|
| Na | 156 | Chloride | 100 |
| Potassium | 3.8 | Glucose | 140 |
| Albumin | 3.6 | Total protein | 8.0 |
| Bicarbonate (HCO3) 27 | | | |
| BUN | 33 | Creatinine | 1.2 |

Urine studies shows

Osmolality   900mosm/kg   Specific gravity   1.035

Urine sodium 95          Urine potassium   45

24 hr urine volume = 800mls

Weight today 44 kg

**What is the free water deficit?**

A   2.4 Liters

B   4.5 Liters

C   6 Liters

D   3 Liters

# ANSWERS

1  Answer E

Review steps in acid base balance

Low PH and low HCO3 **shows metabolic acidosis**

Anion gap is 28 – **anion gap metabolic acidosis**

If corrected HCO3 for anion gap, there is **associated metabolic alkalosis** (corrected HCO3= 28-12 + 22= 40

Using winter formula, the expected PCO2 ( 1.5 x 22 + 8= 41) is lower than  actual PCO2 (50) **= respiratory acidosis**

Thus the patient had combined anion gap metabolic acidosis, metabolic alkalosis and respiratory acidosis




2  Answer C

-Low PH and HCO3 suggest metabolic acidosis, Anion gap is 9

Using the winter formula Expected PCO2( 36.5+ 2) is lower than actual PCO2

**=Non anion gap Metabolic Acidosis from GI loss AND respiratory acidosis**

3  Answer is A

The anion gap is within normal range

Correct answer is Non anion gap metabolic acidosis

4  Answer – D

The high PH and elevated HC03 consistent with metabolic alkalosis
The elevated PC02 shows presence of additional Respiratory acidosis


5  Answer B

An elevated PH and serum HC03 consistent with Metabolic Alkalosis

The elevated urine chloride suggestive of chloride - non responsive
(suspected hyperaldosteronism)


6  Answer D

- The low urine chloride is consistent with Metabolic Alkalosis due to vomiting- chloride responsive
- No additional respiratory disorder


7  Answer B

Calculate the volume of free water needed to correct the hypernatremia
Total body water in this patient

$= 45 \times 0.5$

$= 22.5 \, L$

0.5 of weight is being used here since elderly and female


Free water deficit

$$= \frac{163 - 140}{140} \times \text{Total body water}$$

$$= 23/140 \times 22.5$$

$$= 3.6 \text{ L}$$

Total free water deficit in this patient is 3.6 L.

Note in a clinical scenario, estimate continuous volume loss and add this to the water deficit to estimate total volume needed to replace in the next 24-36 hrs

8 Answer is B

Total body water = 84 × 0.6

$$= 50.4 \text{ L}$$

Free water deficit

$$= \frac{151 - 140}{140} \times \text{Total body water}$$

$$= 11/140 \times 50.4$$

$$= 3.96 \text{ L}$$

Total free water deficit in this patient is 3.9 L.

**9** Answer  A

1 Since low serum bicarbonate level – suggestive either a primary metabolic acidosis or a respiratory alkalosis

2 However the low arterial PH of 7.36 is consistent with an acidosis state.

Thus the patient has **a primary metabolic acidosis**


**10** Answer  A

Since high serum bicarbonate level and high PH

Thus the patient has **a primary metabolic alkalosis**


**11** Correct Answer is A

Presence of acidosis with low HC03 and low PH consistent with metabolic acidosis

Expected PC02 is within expected range of actual PC02
( = 1.5 x Hc03 + 8  ) +/- 2  =  38 which is within 2 of the actual PC02.
So no additional respiratory acidosis or alkalosis


**12** Correct Answer is C

1 Since low serum bicarbonate level – suggestive either a primary metabolic acidosis or a respiratory alkalosis

2 However the low arterial PH of 7.23 is consistent with an acidosis state.

Thus the patient has **a primary metabolic acidosis (hyperchloremic non anion gap acidosis)**

Expected PC02 ( 1.5 x 17 + 8= 33.5) is lower than actual PCO2 suggesting an additional respiratory acidosis

**13** Correct Answer is D

1 Since low serum bicarbonate level – suggestive either a primary metabolic acidosis or a respiratory alkalosis

2 However the low arterial PH of 7.34 is consistent with an acidotic sis state.

Thus the patient has **a primary metabolic acidosis (hyperchloremic non anion gap acidosis)**

Expected PC02 (1.5 x 17 + 8= 33.5) is higher than actual PCO2 (30± 2 )  suggesting an additional respiratory alkalosis

=   Primary metabolic acidosis and respiratory alkalosis

**14** Correct Answer is C

1 Since low serum bicarbonate level – suggestive either a primary metabolic acidosis or a respiratory alkalosis

2 However the low arterial PH of 7.27 is consistent with an acidosis state.

Thus the patient has **a primary metabolic acidosis**

**The elevated expected Actual PC02 (56) more than the expected PC02 (  20 x 1.5 + 8 = 38 ± 2)   shows a combined metabolic and respiratory acidosis**

**17** Correct Answer is D

1 Since low serum bicarbonate level – suggestive either a primary metabolic acidosis or a respiratory alkalosis

2 However the high arterial PH of 7.42 is consistent with an alkalosis state.

Thus the patient has **a primary respiratory alkalosis**


**18** Correct Answer is B

**The presence of hypotension warrant replacement with NS regardless of etiology of Hyponatremia**


**19** Correct Answer is B

Total Sodium deficit = TBW x change in Sodium

$$= 0.55 \times weight \times (135 - 125$$
$$= 0.55 \times 60 \times 10$$
$$= 330 \text{ meq}$$


**20** Correct Answer is A

Water deficit = 154-140/ 140 x TBW

= 14/140 × 0.6 × 84 = 5.04 Liters

**21** Correct Answer is C

-Anion gap metabolic acidosis and a concurrent metabolic alkalosis.

The low serum bicarbonate level and a pH shows metabolic acidosis

The anion gap is 140- (80 + 11) = 49

Δ Anion gap of 49 – 12 = 37

Δ HCO3 = 24 – 11 = 13

Since Δ Anion gap is higher than Δ HCO3 ( or Δ Anion gap + serum HCO3 = 37 + 11 = 48 ) There is concurrent metabolic alkalosis

**22** Answer A

Plasma volume = 0.07 × weight × (1 - Hematocrit)

= 0.07 × 76 × ( 1- 23/100)

= 0.07 × 76 × 0.77

= 4 Liters

**23** Correct answer is A

Using Cockcroft-Gault formular

$$\text{Creatinine clearance} = \frac{140-\text{Age} \times 72}{\text{Weight} \times \text{Creatinine}}$$

$$= \frac{(140-82) \times 72}{82 \times 1.7}$$

$$= 29 \text{ mls/min}$$

## 24 Correct answer is D

In female, and in using the calculation from question 23 above
eGFR = 29 × 0.85 = 25.4 mls/min

## 25 Correct Answer is B

$$FeNa = \frac{\text{Urine Na} \times \text{Serum Cr}}{\text{Serum Na} \times \text{Urine Cr}} \times 100$$

$$= \frac{32 \times 2.5}{136 \times 20}$$

$$= 0.029 \times 100$$

$$= 2.9\%$$

## 26 Correct Answer is A

$$\text{Fractional excretion of Urea} = \frac{\text{Ur Urea} \times \text{Serum Cr}}{\text{Serum Urea(BUN)} \times \text{Urine Cr}} \times 100$$

$$= \frac{140 \times 2.5}{56 \times 20}$$

$$= 31.25\%$$

**27  Correct Answer is A.**

The presence of diuretics increase sodium excretion and can give a calculated FeNa >2% even in the presence of pre-renal azotemia

**28  Correct Answer is A**

**Free water deficit-** $= TBW \times (156 - 140)/140$

$= (44 \times 0.5) \times 16/140$

$= 22 \times 0.11$

$= 2.5\ L$

The above is the water deficit. This need to be slowly over 24 – 48 hrs not exceeding decrease in serum sodium of 12meq/day in order to minimize risk of cerebral edema from rapid rate of correction

- This is done usually by replacing half the total water deficit in 24 hrs and the other half over another 24 hrs

**Ideally then Calculate the additional ongoing urine water loss by Fractional** excretion of electrolytes free water FEW

FEW = ( 1 - urine Na + K/ serum Na) x 24 hr urine volume

$$= \left(1 - \frac{95 + 45}{156}\right) \times 800cc$$

$$= 1 - 140/156 \times 0.8$$
$$= (1-0.89) \times 0.8 = 0.11 \times 0.8$$
$$= 0.08 \text{ L or } 80 \text{ cc}$$

Thus total free water need to replace = obligatory free water + free water deficit

In the first 24 hrs - Total water volume needed = 24 hr obligatory water loss + water deficit/ 2

$$= 80 \text{ cc} + 2500/2$$
$$= 80 + 1250$$
$$= 1330 \text{mls}$$

Acknowledgment

Thanks to Ese, Larry, Greg, Moriamo and Vivian for all your help

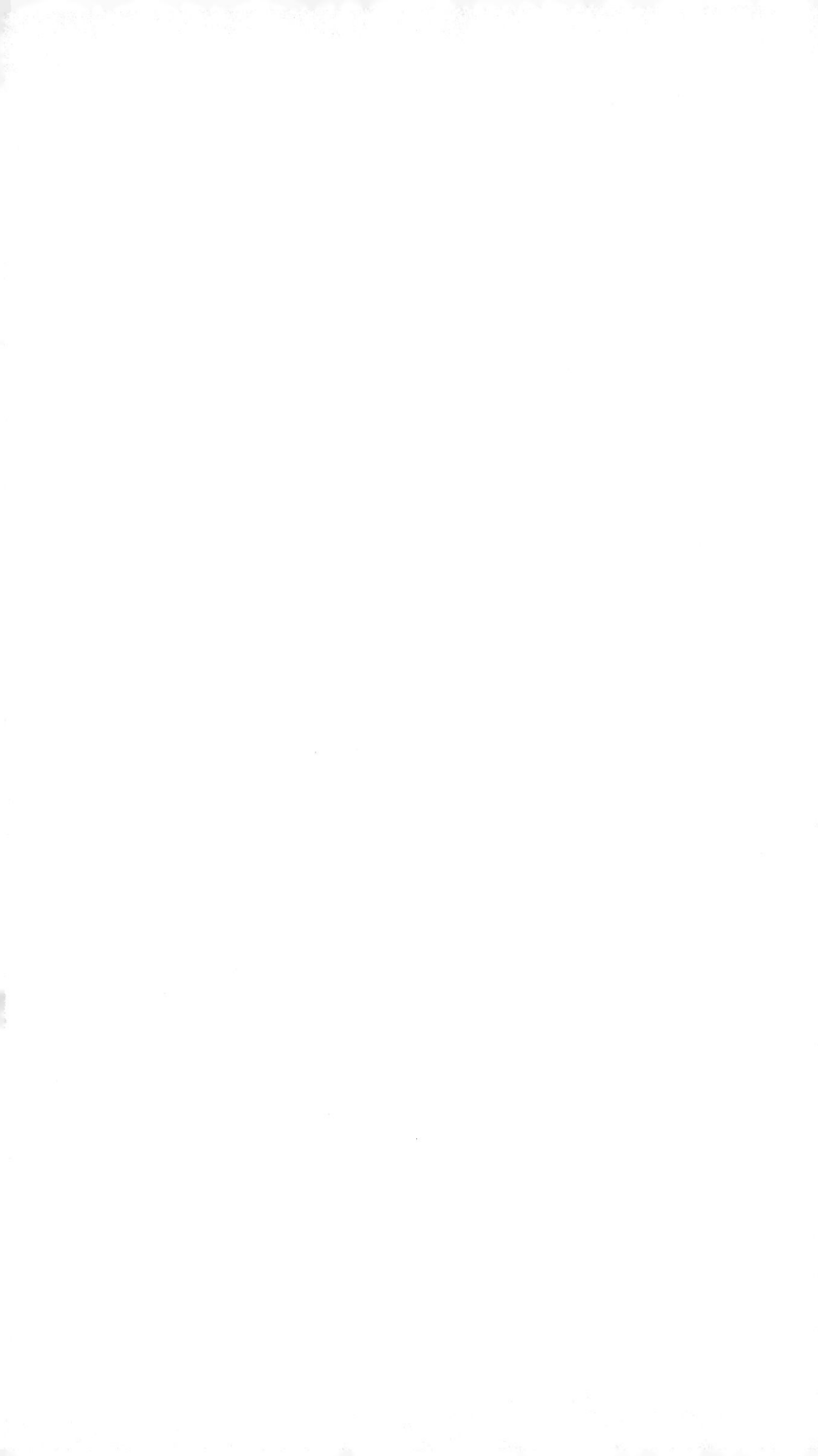

www.ingramcontent.com/pod-product-compliance
Lightning Source LLC
Chambersburg PA
CBHW030818180526
45163CB00003B/1331